# MINDFULNESS EXERCISES FOR BEGINNERS

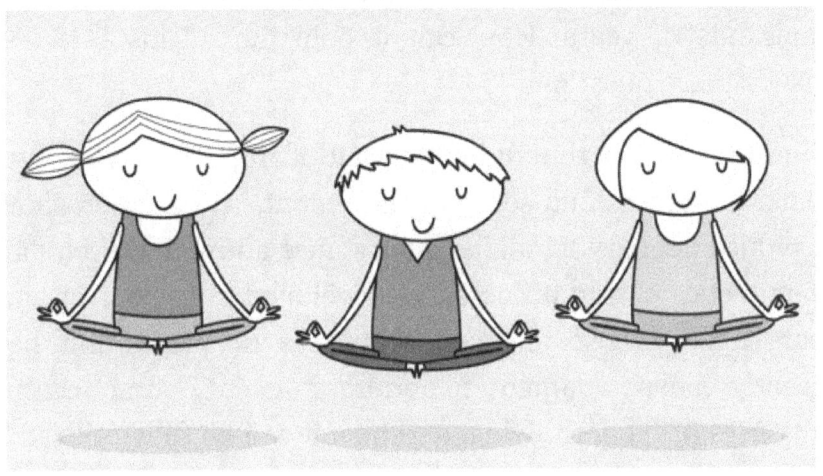

## By: Patricia A Carlisle

# Introduction

I want to thank you and congratulate you for choosing the book, ***"MIDEFULNESS EXERCISES FOR BEGINNERS"***.

This book contains proven steps and strategies on how to be mindful to help improve your well-being and live a better life.

What is this thing called mindfulness...Has it been around for thousands of years...How can it help me? This book will answer these questions.

Mindfulness is a time-honored way of improving your well-being, happiness and sense of fulfillment. It has been shown to reduce depression, anxiety, substance abuse and even pain. The practice of mindfulness was developed in India over 2500 years ago. These ancient techniques of meditation have recently been adapted to address twenty first century pressures of modern living, and how it can be fully utilized by beginners.

Have you ever felt a little down, maybe upset about what someone said to you, or perhaps anxious about a meeting in a few days' time? Possibly you've found your thoughts running out of control, or you worry a lot. Maybe you have a serious disease, in pain, or suffering from a mental illness such as depression or schizophrenia? Mindfulness may help in all these situations.

Thanks again for choosing this book, I hope you enjoy it!

# TABLE OF CONTENT

# Chapter 1

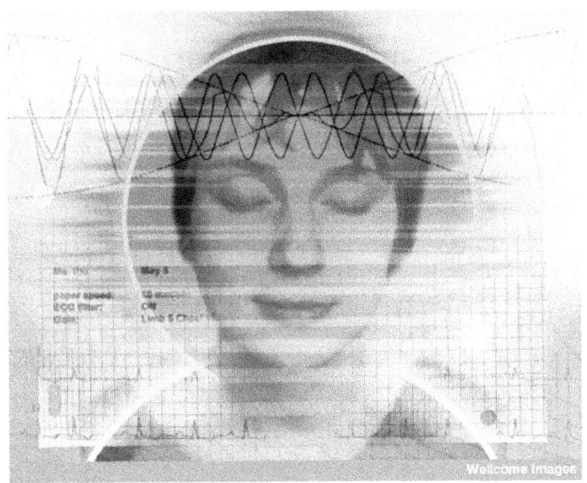

## WHAT IS MINDFULNESS

So what does it mean to be mindful? As a child I was occasionally told, -Mind your manners! This mean I should be aware of what I was doing, and how it was affecting other people-usually adults! That's not a bad start; mindfulness certainly is about paying attention. Paying attention to what is happening right now, right before our eyes-and ears and nose, and other senses, including our internal ones. Also, what pains and tensions are there in our body, how are you feeling right now, are you aware of what you are thinking, or are you on automatic, daydreaming, or perhaps going over and over a difficult encounter?

Many of the problems mentioned above relate to the future or the past. Anxiety and stress can result from worrying about future events. Depression is often associated with replaying past events in our mind. We go over past events, or we are anxious about the future. Much of our thinking is not in the present, and the present is the only time we've got-a series of present moments. By moving our life more into the present moment, we relate to the past and the future in a different way, and our habitual unhelpful thinking about past and future events drops away, becomes less insistent, and we find right here, right now a more vibrant and alive place to be.

Since I've been practicing mindfulness, I've regained a lot of the energy spent fighting off sadness and anger, my mind is much clearer now, said one client. The flowers seem brighter, said another, with a puzzled expression on her face.

Turing in to the present moment were sensations come in-a sensation is always in the present. Feel your legs and buttocks pressing on the chair for a few seconds...listen carefully to any sound nearby. Happily, you have just been practicing mindfulness! By doing mindfulness exercises based around sensations (e.g. the breath), and by becoming more aware in our daily life of what's going on around us, we can spend more time in the present.

# Chapter 2

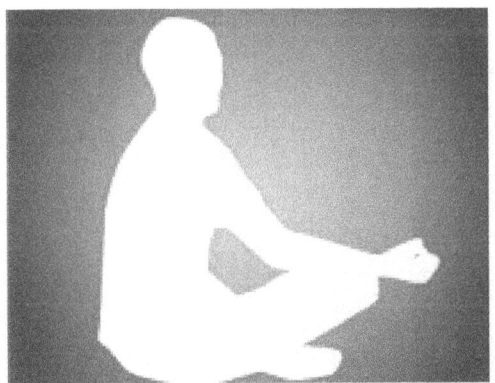

## WHAT'S MOST IMPORTANT ABOUT MINDFULNESS

OVER THE CENTURIES, mindfulness exercise has developed a vast reservoir of knowledge about the mind. Especially as we begin to learn meditation, all the suggestions and ideas may feel overwhelming. It's best to keep our practice simple. Set attainable goals, and strive for them with positive energy. Don't worry about difficulties, but instead feel glad about any benefits that come. Even negative experiences, or so-called shortcomings can be a benefit if we view them positively.

When meditating, we should relax and let go, rather than chasing our worries and desires. We usually sit down to meditate, but much of what we learn about meditation can be carried into all our daily activities. Words are necessary to describe how to meditate, and how to bring the right attitude to our lives. However, the important thing is to practice and feel, without being overly concerned about concepts, categories, or rules. Be patient and open, and work with what your own life brings you.

# Chapter 3

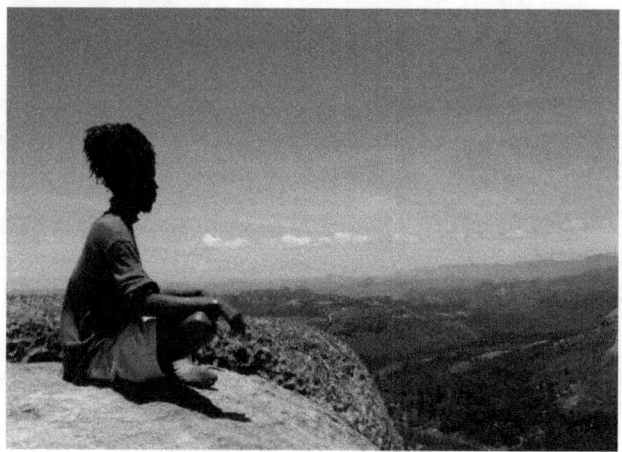

## THE BEST PLACE TO PRACTICE

The best place to practice mindfulness training and healing is a peaceful, pleasant place where there are few distractions, where the mind can be calm and the body comfortable, and where we can feel alert, spacious, and happy. Stages of the past have praised a variety of places, depending on the character of the beginner, the practice, and the season.

Among the favored solitary locations are those that have a clear, far reaching view, like the top of a sky-kissing mountain, or the lap of a prosperous field. Some beginners have ageless song of joy, and playing free from fear. Others suggest training by the ocean with its dancing, ever-changing waves, or a river with its mighty, natural flow. Still others have trained in the dry caves of empty valleys where there is an atmosphere of sublime peace. If we do not live in such natural settings, we should find a pleasant place in our own home space, make the best of it, and rejoice.

Choose the quietest room or corner of a room of your home, during a time when there will be few disturbances from the telephone, children, roommates, spouse, or friends. Then feel good; good about the place, the time, and the opportunity to have this place and time. Arouse joy at this chance to realize that study mindfulness of your life.

Generally, it is better for beginners to practice alone, in a place that presents no obstructions. After gaining strength in the training, we can seek harder situations that require more tolerance and discipline-with obstacles such as disturbances from people or noise from traffic- to strengthen ourselves in using the hardships that come our way.

Finally, when we are ready, we can practice dwelling in the worst situations, with all kinds of mental temptation and emotional turmoil. By practicing diligently in this way, eventually we will be able to face, and transform any situation into a source of strength without losing our peaceful mind. Wherever we live will then become a palace of enlightenment and purity. Every event will be a teaching. After that the place won't matter; the only need will be to choose a place where we can best serve others.

# Chapter 4

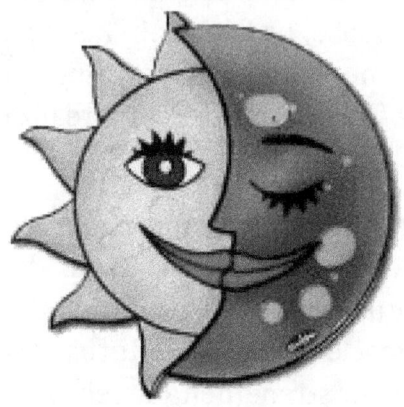

## CHOOSING A TIME

Although any time is fine for training, peace and calm are helpful for a beginner. Early morning is good, for then the day itself is fresh and the mind is clear. However, some might feel relaxed and ready to meditate in the evening. Choose a time, observe it regularly, and be happy with it. If you can, allow nothing to interfere with your regular practice.

Whatever meditation or healing exercise we do, we should give ourselves to it. We should not dream about the future or make plans in our heads. Do not run after the past or grasp at the present. All kinds of thoughts or mental experiences may arise during meditation, but instead of grasping at them, let them come and go. Practice every day. Even if we meditate for a short time, the consistency will keep the contemplative experience alive, and steady us on the path of healing.

How long should we meditate? Your mind is the healer, so the answer depends on your needs and abilities. You could meditate for a few minutes, for twenty minutes, or for an hour. You could meditate for many hours, with rest periods, over a long period of time. Don't be overly concerned with time, but rather consider what feels right. It's especially good to practice when we are happy, healthy, and relatively free of problems. Then, when we face suffering-which will certainly come-we will have the skillful means ready to apply. When we are in the midst of pain and confusion, we may have less clarity, energy, and opportunity for training.

# Chapter 5

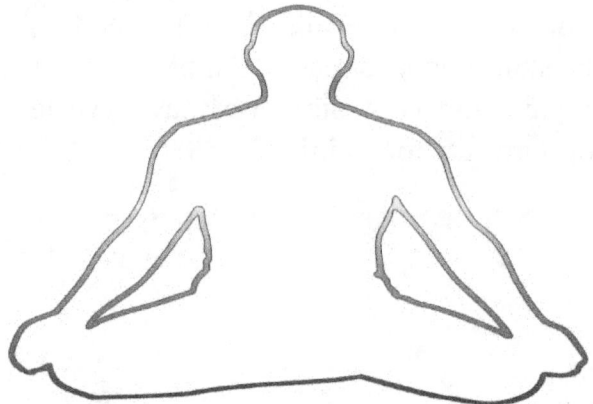

## POSTURE

The essential goal of any of the various postures for meditating is to relax the muscles, and open the channels in the body so that energy and breath can flow naturally through them. Whatever posture makes our body straight and relaxed, but not stiff, will produce a natural flow of energy, and allow the mind to be calm and flexible. The purpose of the physical postures is summarized in this popular.

## Tibetan saying:

- If your body is straight, your channels will be straight.

- If your channels are straight, your mind will be straight.

One of the most popular Buddhist meditation positions is called the lotus posture, in which one sits cross-legged on the floor with the right foot on the left thigh and the left foot on the right thigh. Most Westerners find the half-lotus easier, with one ankle resting on the fold of the opposite leg. If you sit on a small cushion, your torso will be raised up a bit in a way that you may find is open and relaxed. Your hands are placed on your lap, right hand over left with tips on thumbs touching, and palms up. The elbows should be slightly away from the body, in a natural, wing like position, instead of being cramped or pressed inward.

The chin is lowered to allow the neck to bend slightly, so that it feels natural to focus the eyes a yard or two in front, at the level of the tip of the nose. The tip of the tongue is gently touching the upper palate. The most important element of all is to keep the spine straight. Some people may find this posture very difficult if they have back problems. You may want to sit on a chair to meditate, but make sure the chair allows you to keep your spine straight rather than slumping.

Whatever posture you choose, remember that the purpose is not to be uncomfortable. You should be comfortable enough so that your mind can relax and concentrate. It's best to meditate in a sitting posture, our mind is capable of healing wherever we are, and under any circumstance, as long as we are aware.

# Chapter 6

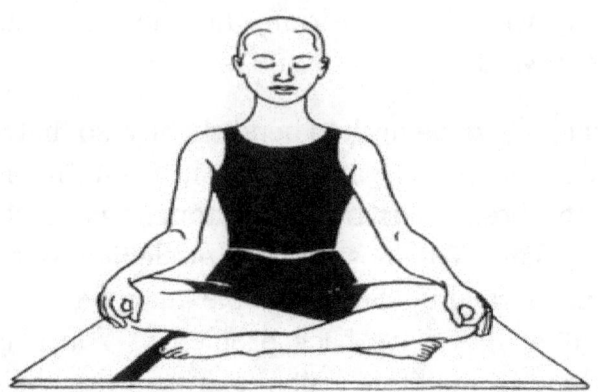

## RELAXATION

To release the struggles of our mind-the conceptual and emotional pressures that grip us-we should relax the tightness of our muscles when we meditate. If tension is gathered anywhere in your muscles, bring awareness to the area and release the tightness. Relaxation provides a calm atmosphere in which we can light the candle of healing energy.

However, relaxation does not mean indulging in a lazy, careless, semiconscious, or sleepy state of mind. At times we may need to rest and be sleepy, but the most effective meditation is awake, alert and clear. This is the way to touch our peaceful, joyous nature. Allow yourself to stay relaxed in the transition from meditation back to your daily routine. Get up slowly, and ease your mind into your activities. This way, you bring a spacious mind into your life.

# Chapter 7

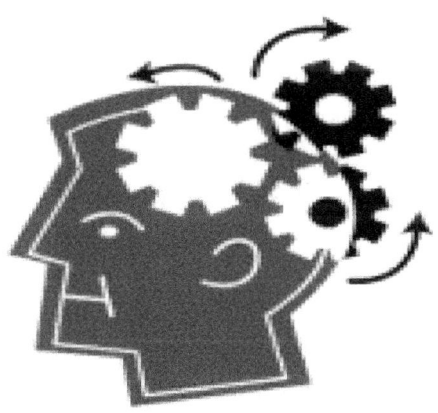

## CREATING MENTAL SPACE

Few of us give ourselves completely to what we are doing. We bring our job problems home, and so we have no chance to enjoy our home life. Then we take our home problems to work and cannot devote ourselves to our job. While trying to meditate, we fondle our mental images and feelings, which give us no real chance to concentrate. We end up having no life to live because we always dwell to the past or future. If we cluttered up our homes with too much furniture, we would have no place to live. If our minds are cluttered with plans, concerns, thoughts, and emotional patterns, we have no space for our true selves. Many people feel their lives are too crowded to meditate.

Even when they have time at home to meditate, they feel too distracted. To bring our full attention and energy to our home lives, and to meditation, we need mental space. We can consciously create space for ourselves. We can decide to leave our worries about work behind us. If it is helpful, we could visualize these worries in the form of papers and computers that are safely back in the office.

We could even imagine borderlines separating our work lives from home. Or, we could create a protective tent of energy or light in our minds, enclosing us in our home, and granting complete privacy for what we are doing now. Meditation can be a haven of warmth and space, but we may feel resistance to meditating or think of it as a chore. One way to create an open and relaxed feeling is to go back to the atmosphere of childhood. Since childhood, we have learned and experienced a lot of wonderful things in this generous world.

However, it is easy to be caught reaching a stage where we suffocate ourselves with our own views, feelings, habits, and reactions. Thinking back, we remember as children a day seemed to last for a long time, more like the way we experience a month now. A year was so long there was no end to it. Gradually our perception changed. Our preoccupations, concepts, and attachments grew day by day. Now the open space is no longer there in our minds. As we grew, we felt time become shorter and shorter, and now a year passes in the blink of an eye. It is not because time actually becomes shorter, but because we do not have the mental space to feel open and free. We run around at full speed, and crowd our minds with a houseful of thoughts, concepts, and emotions. When our minds are calm, we feel every minute of time, but if your minds chase after everything going on around us, we feel that the day has ended before it has even begun.

# CHAPTER 8

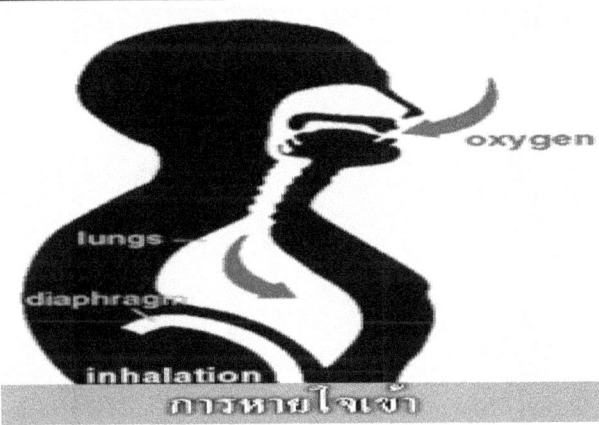

## BREATHING

In any kind of meditation, it is important to breathe naturally and calmly. Contemplation of our breathing, the mind's awareness of the breath, in and out, is in itself a foundation for realizing our true nature. Highly experienced mediators use this approach as a means to realize selflessness; it is a good way to calm ourselves, focus our minds, and establishes a flow of energy that enables healing to progress.

At the beginning, you may feel it is impossible to concentrate fully on the simple act of breathing in and out. It can be shocking to see how fast the mind moves. Do not worry about the coming and going of thoughts or images. Gently being your consciousness back to your breathing, and give your awareness completely to this. By just allowing our minds to touch and unite with the natural process of breathing, we can release stress, and feel more relaxed.

Awareness of breathing is also a very powerful method to release any difficult emotion that has us in a viselike grip. As we'll wee in the healing exercises, a particularly helpful technique is to concentrate on your relaxed exhalations.  In this way, gasping is relaxed.

# CHAPTER 9

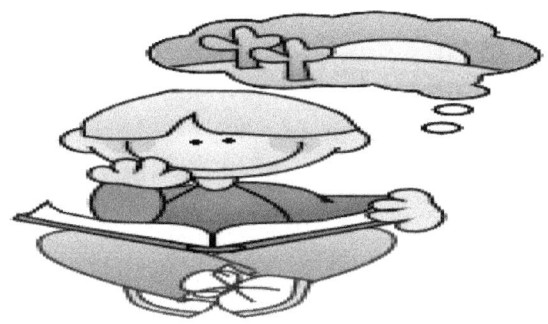

## VISUALIZATION

One of the best tools in exercising the mind is visualization, which can transform our mental patterns from negative to positive. Some beginners at meditation regard visualization as a difficult or unusual mental activity. Actually, it is quite natural, for we think in images all the time. When we think of our friends or family, or imagine ourselves at a lovely beach, or mountain like, we see these images in our minds quite vividly.

In meditation we visualize for a particular purpose, but the mental process is the same. With practice, we can get better at it. Although visualization has a long heritage in Tibetan Buddhist practice, people who have no knowledge of or interest in Buddhism have found the technique extremely helpful.

For instance, some professional athletes visualize improving their performance and realizing their full potential. Positive images inspire all sorts of people in all kinds of activities. I know of a music teacher from Cleveland who overcame stage fright using her own improvised approach. Although she's a trained singer with a splendid voice, she dreaded her weekly duties as the cantor at a local synagogue.

One Sabbath before the service, she wept so violently that she suddenly realized how crippling her fears had become. That's when she made up her mind to enjoy herself instead! To help herself do this, she sat somewhere quiet and imagined herself leading the prayer successfully, singing in a way that felt good to her, but without being overly worried about the melodies that had been difficult in practice.

She imagined what it would be like to be very confident about her singing. In her mind, she heard the beautiful sound of her own voice, giving delight to the congregation. She envisioned the whole scene of the prayer service, and felt a lovely, expansive sense of gladness and inspiration at being able to share the music with everyone. She now is happy in her singing, and is not bothered if she feels a bit nervous ahead of time.

And, when she teaches, she suggests to her music students that they also use their imagination to learn how to be more relaxed and bring joy to their singing. In meditation, it's best to keep your eyes open or partly open, in order to stay awake, and in this world. However, it may be helpful for some beginners to close their eyes at first. The most important point in visualizing is to call up the positive image and warmth, and whole-heartedness. Give your full attention to the mental object, become totally absorbed in it.

Allow the mind and the object to become one. I few see the image in our minds half-heartedly, or in a distracted way, our concentration is limited. Then as if we were staring blankly at an object just with our eyes, instead of with our whole being. "Abiding in contemplation' has to develop in the mind, not in the senses such as the eyes."

For beginners especially, the key is to feel the presence of what you are imagining. Your visualization doesn't need to be elaborate or detailed; the clarity and stability of your mental images are what matters.

# CHAPTER 10

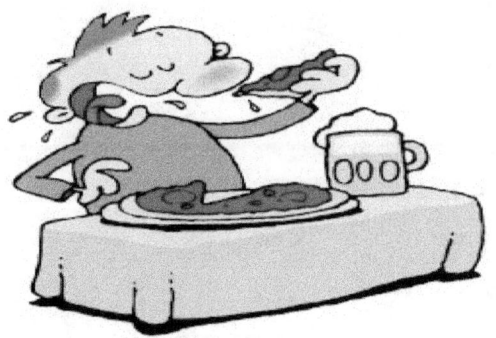

## MINDFULNESS OF EATING

Before you choose what you will be eating, come to a place of mindfulness: Sense what your body needs. Notice whether saliva production increases as you look at the platter. Take your time to choose one thing.

Focus with clear awareness on each movement, and each moment of the experience as you move your arm and hand and fingers towards the object, and pick it up place it on the palm of your hand, or hold it between your fingers.

Imagine you have just come to Earth and awakened to this substance you have not encountered before. Explore it with all your senses as if you have never seen it before. Scan it; explore every part of it with your eyes as it sits on your palm or in your fingers. Turn it around. Notice the texture, the light on it, its shape; whether it is soft, hard, coarse, smooth. Notice any thoughts that arise (like "why am I doing this?"), And see if you can just notice the thoughts and let them be...before bringing your awareness back to the object.

Take the food beneath your nose, and carefully notice the smell of it. Bring the food to one ear and squeeze it, roll it, listen for any sound coming from it. Begin to slowly bring the food to your mouth, noticing that the arm knows exactly where to go and perhaps noticing your mouth watering. Gently place the food in your mouth, or take one bit if it is larger than one bit-size, but do not chew yet. Feel it on your tongue; its weight, temperature, size, texture. Explore the sensations of it in your mouth.

When you are ready, as beginner you will intentionally bite into it. Does it go automatically to one side of the mouth? Notice when the taste releases. Slowly, slowly chew, noticing the change in consistency, until you are conscious of the impulse to swallow. Sense the food moving down to your throat, and into your esophagus on its way to your stomach. Sit with the experience, noticing any vestiges remaining in your mouth, on your tongue, any taste, feelings...satisfaction, pleasure, aversion.

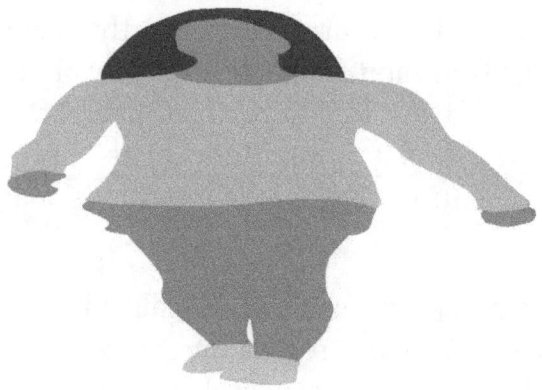

# CHAPTER 11

## MINDFULNESS OF WALKING

Before you start, prepare the space. Removing your shoes is good, if that's possible. And find a place where you can walk for about 12-14 steps before you have to turn. Now first notice your body as you stand in stillness. Feel the connection of the body to the ground, or the floor. Become aware of your surroundings, taking in any sights, smells, tastes, sounds, or other sensations. Notice any thoughts or emotions, and let them be. Notice your arms by your sides, or if you prefer, hold your right hand in your left hand at the front, or clasp your hands at your back.

Notice your breath, moving in and out of your body. No need to change it; just let it be. Now shift your weight to the left leg, and begin to lift your right foot up. Move it forward, place it back down on the ground. Mindfully shift the weight the right leg, and begin to lift the lift foot up, move it forward, and place it back down on the ground. And continue with this walking...walking mindfully, walking slowly, and paying attention to the sensations on the soles of your feet. As each part of the sole, form heel to toe, touches the ground. Lifting, moving, placing, Lifting, moving, and placing. Notice how the body moves as you walk. Walk with awareness, one step at a time.

When it is time to turn, maintain the flow of mindfulness, and bring your awareness to the intricate process of turning. Slowly, and with attention to each movement necessary to turn, begin to walk back to where you started. One step at a time. Lifting, moving, and placing. Lifting, moving, and placing. Find a rhythm that suits you. That suits your body and your balance. As you move forward, notice your body, notice your head sitting on your shoulders, your arms & hands, your torso, your legs, moving you forward, step by step. Notice any thoughts that arise and let them be. Returning your focus to the sensation of walking, Lifting, moving, placing.

Notice your breath. Has it moved into a rhythm; a rhythm that fits with your pace of walking, step by step? There's no need to change your breathing, but you might find that it has changed without you noticing it. Continue walking, taking care of notice each intricate movement required at the turns, one step at a time. Practice this for a moment. And next time you return to your starting place, be still. Notice the sensations in your body; bring awareness to your breath. Notice the stillness when movement ceases. And appreciate the time you have spent today, practicing mindfulness of walking. These simple practices are major for the beginner.

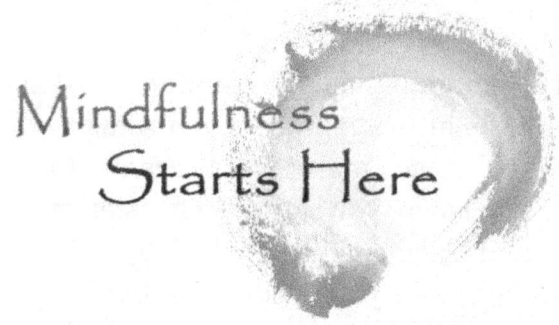

# CHAPTER 12

## OPENESSS AND MINDFULNESS

One way to break through the feeling of emotional suffocation is to go someplace high where you can have a far-reaching view, such as the top of a mountain or a building. If the sky is very clear, sit with your back to the sun. Concentrate on the depth of the open sky without moving your eyes. Slowly exhale, and experience the openness, vastness, and validness.

Feel that the whole universe has become one in the vast openness. Think that all phenomena-trees, mountains, and rivers-have dissolved spontaneously into the open sky. Your mind and body have dissolved there too. All have vanished like clouds disappearing from the sky. Relax in the feeling of openness, free from boundaries and limitations.

This exercise is not only effective for calming the mind, but can also generate higher realization. If you cannot go to such a place, choose any spot from which you have a good view of the sky, or from which you can at least visualize the open sky.

# CHAPTER 13

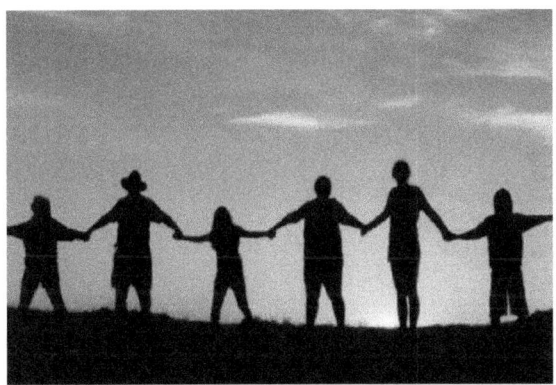

## MERGING WITH ONENESS

Merging with oneness means being one with whatever we are experiencing. It sometimes helps in the beginning to describe oneness in words: for example, it is like being a swimmer at one with the vast ocean.

But actually words are not necessary for the experience of oneness and openness. We simply let go of our struggles and relax no need to put labels such as "good" or "bad" on experiences. We drop expectations about how we should feel or want to feel, and instead allow ourselves to be with the feeling or to go within it.

By merging with experiences or feelings, the character of experience can change. By allowing ourselves to be just as we are in the present moment, the walls of our discriminations and sensitivities will soften, or fall away altogether. Our minds and hearts open, and our energy flows. This is a powerful healing.

# CHAPTER 14

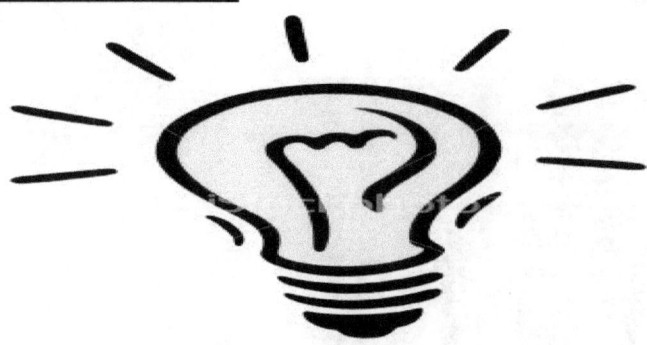

## ENLIGHTENED ATTITUDE

We should develop the attitude that "I am doing this mindfulness training for the service, happiness, benefit, and enlightenment of all beings," or, "I am training in order to make myself a proper tool to serve and fulfill the needs of all beings." In the scriptures this is call the enlightened attitude. This intention to dedicate our training to others in a powerful way, and to open our closed, restricted hearts, will produces a strong spiritual energy-a blessing-and sows in us the seed of enlightenment.

If we develop and maintain this "enlightenment mind," then whatever we do will spontaneously become a mindful training, and means of benefit for all. Even for someone who is not religious, it will be very helpful to reflect upon his or her link to family, friends, community, and all people everywhere, instead of pursuing training merely for selfish goals.

Opening to compassion can be difficult, and we can be subject to negative emotions and attitudes. However, the intention itself is important. By developing compassion, the stream of merit can flow day and night, and lead us to full realization of our true nature.

# CHAPTER 15

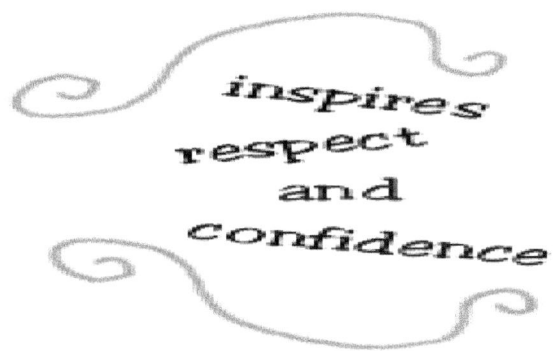

*inspires respect and confidence*

## CONFIDENCE/ PERCEPTION

CONFIDENCE IS our best ally as we learn how to train our minds and tap into our strengths. We need confidence in ourselves and in the path we are following.

If we don't have this, our half-committed minds may not even achieve a half-baked result. Many of us lack self-confidence. We feel hopeless and unfulfilled-too weak to strive for any higher goal. Lack of confidence can result from mental character or upbringing. If it is our mental character, this can be harder to change, but if it is our upbringing that has stunted our growth, it is not so difficult to change and grow.

PURE PERCEPTION, the habit of seeing things as positive or negative is created in our minds. The chain of emotions in our minds-like and dislike, craving and hatred-produce more pain or craving.

The way to transform our habitual reactions is to bring a positive attitude to every situation, and feel the positive energy deeply. Pure perception means to see everything as pure, perfect, peaceful, joyful, and enlightened. In our everyday lives, it may appear to us that we are burdened by troubles.

However, the Buddhist view is troubles, in their ultimate nature, are like waves on the surface of the ocean. A storm may toss the waves on the surface, but the ocean below remains calm.

We can find peace within a difficult experience, and see something as positive, even if it is raging in its surface manifestation. If we see something as peaceful, even thought it appears to be strongly negative.

# Conclusion

Thank you again for choosing this book!

I hope this book was able to help you to be mindful in your life.

The next step is to consciously recognize the peaceful feeling in our minds and rest within that experience.

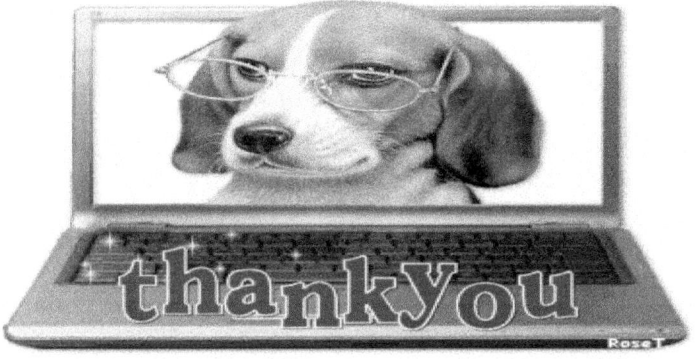

Finally, if you enjoyed this book would you be kind enough to share your experience and leave a review for this book on Amazon? It'd be greatly appreciated!

Thank you and good luck!

# Preview Of 'OVER 600 Positive Affirmations that will change your Life'

## INTRODUCTION

Where did I get these affirmations? I have read affirmations on prolificliving.com and loved it and thought it would serve as a breather from the discussion that my client's and I have on mental health issue. Affirmations has always put my clients in deep thought and put a smile on their faces. So I put together some of PROLIFICLIVING.COM and my own affirmations for them to enjoy. Please feel free to change the wording to adopt it as yours. I have seen how positive affirmations work in my life as well as my friends and I wanted to share them with you.

It is said, "Affirmations work best in the PRESENT tense, and when you say them consciously and preferably loudly (if the circumstance permits!), and it will help you to adopt positive BELIEVING as well as positive thinking as you embrace these words in the situations that arise in your life." The spoken word plays a big part when it comes to designing our futures. I truly believe we influence the universe word by word. Whatever we speak, it will respond. When we speak a sound, we emit a sound wave into the universe. This sound wave has the ability to cut through the air and becomes a real object. "It therefore exists in our world, intangible and invisible." No words are empty words, because every word we speak can bring energy towards or against us. If you constantly say "I can't," the energy of your words will repel the universal force against you. But if you say "I can!" the universe will give you the abilities to do just that. So speak away; relinquish your fears and remove your anger, predict your own future and live up to your potential with the affirmations that will change your life:

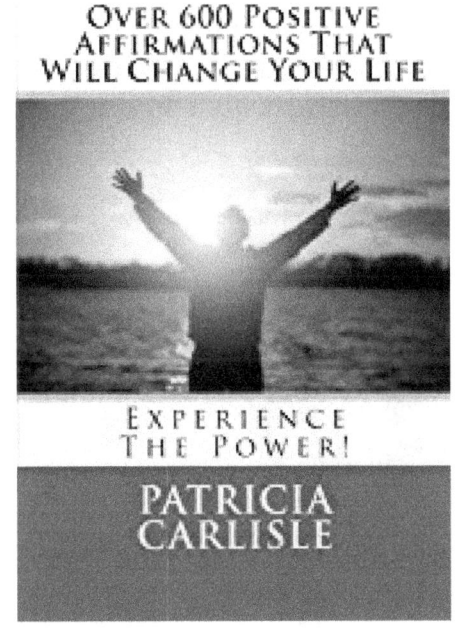

**To read more affirmations, go to**

**amazon .com**

# Check Out My Other Books

Below you'll find some of my other popular books that are popular on Amazon and Kindle as well. Go to Amazon.com to check them out. Alternatively, you can visit my author page on Amazon to see other work done by me.

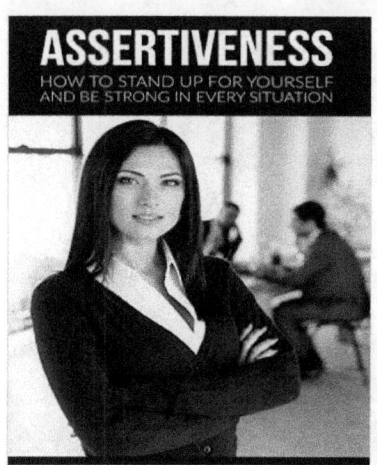

**ASSERTIVENESS: HOW TO STAND UP FOR YOURSELF AND BE STRONG IN EVERY SITUATION.**

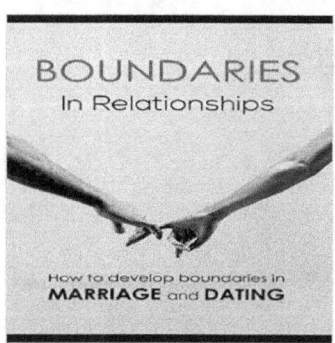

**BOUNDARIES IN RELATIONSHIPS: HOW TO DEVELOP BOUNDARIES IN MARRIAGE AND DATING.**

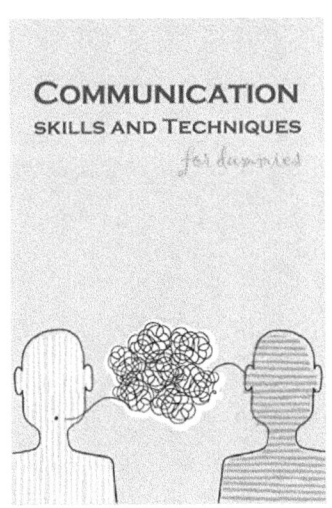

**COMMUNICATION SKILLS AND TECHNIQUES FOR DUMMIES.**

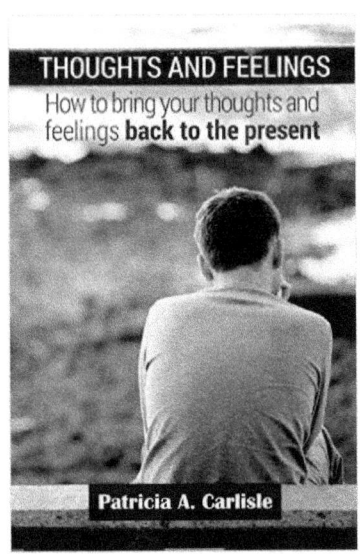

**THOUGHTS AND FEELINGS: HOW TO BRING YOUR THOUGHTS AND FEELINGS BACK TO THE PRESENT.**

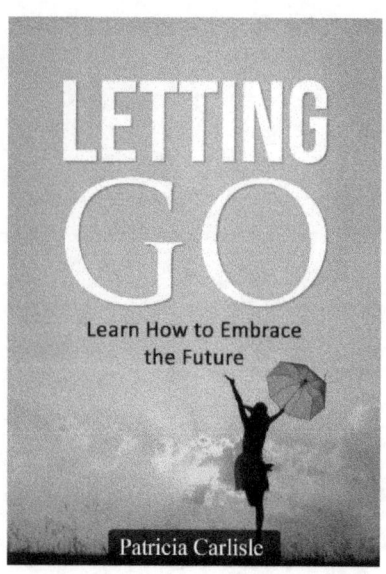

**LETTING GO: LEARN HOW TO EMBRACE THE FUTURE.**

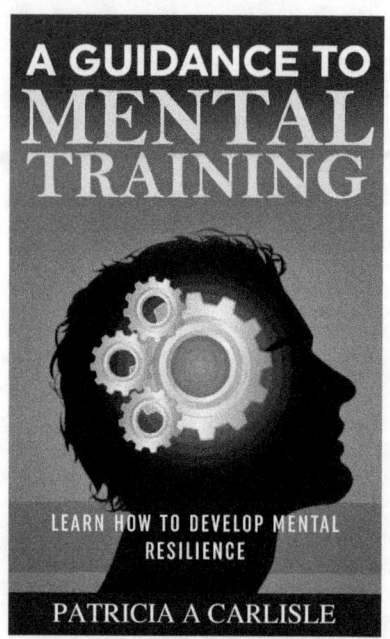

**A GUIDANCE TO MENTAL TRAINING: LEARN HOW TO DEVELOP MENTAL RESILIENCE.**

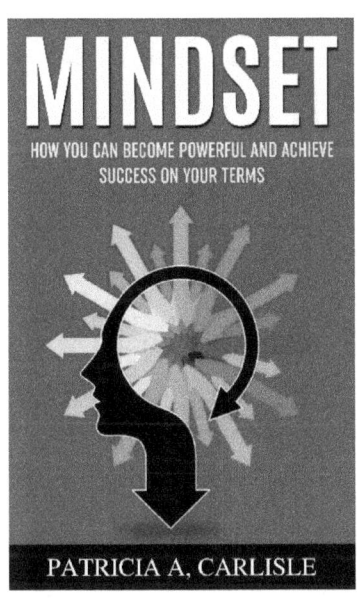

**MINDSET: HOW YOU CAN BECOME POWERFUL AND ACHIEVE SUCCESS ON YOUR TERMS.**

PATRICIA A. CARLISLE

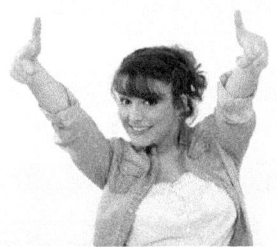

**INSECURE: STOP THE INSECURITY AND LEARN HOW TO OVERCOME JEALOUSY AND BUILD SELF-ESTEEM.**

# BONUS: SUBSCRIBE TO THE FREE BOOK

## Beginners Guide to Yoga & Meditation

"Stressed out? Do You Feel Like The World Is Crashing Down Around You? Want To Take A Vacation That Will Relax Your Mind, Body And Spirit? Well this Easy To Read Step By Step

E-Book Makes It All Possible!"

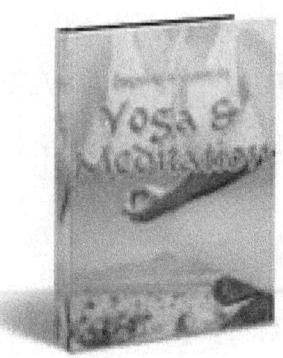

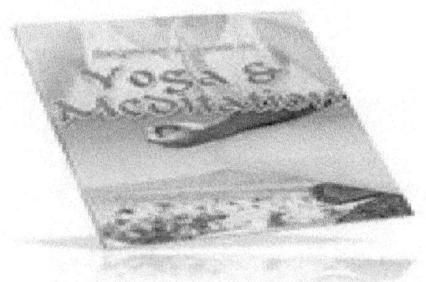

Instructions on how to join our mailing list, and receive a free copy of "Yoga and Meditation" can be found in any of my Kindle eBooks.

# NOTES

# NOTES

# NOTES

# NOTES

# NOTES

# NOTES

# NOTES

# NOTES